DRINKING PROBLEMS

KV-014-048

OTHER BOOKS IN THE SERIES

1. McKenna You — After Childbirth
2. Laidlaw Epilepsy Explained
3. Meadow Help for Bedwetting
4. Illingworth Your Child's Development in the First Five Years
5. Farquhar The Diabetic Child
6. Illingworth Infections — and Immunisation of Your Child
7. Lewis High Blood Pressure
8. Hampton All About Heart Attacks
9. Tattersall Diabetes — a Practical Guide for Patients on Insulin
10. Farquhar Diabetes in Your Teens
11. Chamberlain Pregnancy Questions Answered
12. Ebner Relaxation and Exercise for Childbirth
13. Porter Understanding Back Pain
14. Moll Arthritis and Rheumatism
15. Milner Asthma in Childhood
16. Clark Adult Asthma
17. Heatley Constipation, Piles and other Bowel Disorders
18. Feneley Incontinence

IN PREPARATION

Wood Infertility
Goldberg Depression
Martin Hearing Loss
Thomas Diet and Diabetes
Crisp Anorexia Nervosa
Young Guide to Cancer
Bergman Caring for an Elderly Relative

DRINKING PROBLEMS

Patient Handbook 19

INFORMATION AND ADVICE FOR THE INDIVIDUAL,
FAMILY AND FRIENDS.

JO CHICK MA, DSA, DSW

JONATHAN CHICK MA, MPhil, MRCP, MRCPsych
Royal Edinburgh Hospital, Edinburgh

Churchill Livingstone 🏛

EDINBURGH LONDON MELBOURNE AND NEW YORK 1984

CHURCHILL LIVINGSTONE
Medical Division of Longman Group Limited

Distributed in the United States of America by Churchill
Livingstone Inc., 1560 Broadway, New York, N.Y. 10036,
and by associated companies, branches and representatives
throughout the world.

© Longman Group Limited 1984

All rights reserved. No part of this publication may be
reproduced, stored in a retrieval system, or transmitted in
any form or by any means, electronic, mechanical,
photocopying, recording or otherwise, without the prior
permission of the publishers (Churchill Livingstone, Robert
Stevenson House, 1-3 Baxter's Place, Leith Walk, Edinburgh
EH1 3AF).

First published 1984

ISBN 0 443 02801 X

British Library Cataloguing in Publication Data

Chick, Jo
    Drinking problems.—(Churchill Livingstone
    patient handbook)
    1. Alcoholism
    I. Title   II. Chick, Jonathan
    362.2'92   HV5035

Library of Congress Cataloging in Publication Data

Chick, Jo
    Drinking problems.
    (Churchill Livingstone patient handbook ; 18)
    1. Alcoholism. 2. Alcoholics — Family relationships.
I. Chick, Jonathan. II. Title. III. Series.
HV5035.C48   1984   362.2'92   83-18872

Printed in Singapore by
Huntsmen Offset Printing Pte Ltd.

CONTENTS

1. Is this book for me? 1
2. What is a drinking problem? 4
3. Can anyone develop a drinking problem? 16
4. How are women affected? 21
5. Should I change my drinking pattern? 24
6. How to succeed 30
7. Coping with worry, tension and depression 42
8. How is the family affected? 52
9. How can I help him? 57
10. Marriage and the sexual relationship 65
11. Can friends or colleagues help? 71
12. Going for advice 73
13. Surely it's not that easy? 81
Appendix: addresses of agencies offering help 83

ACKNOWLEDGEMENTS

We owe a great debt to numerous colleagues and friends and above all to our patients and their families for sharing their experiences with us. Thanks for the cartoons to WEEF, Peter Joyce and PUNCH.

1. IS THIS BOOK FOR ME?

We hope this book will help people with drinking problems, and those who are worried about their drinking or who have friends or relatives who complain about it. The book is intended also to be of use to the family and friends of problem drinkers.

'I'm fed-up hearing good advice', say some problem drinkers. They feel they have been nagged enough: 'I can't see what everyone is worried about'. Or perhaps they see there is a problem, but 'people don't realise how difficult it is for me to change my drinking — it's such an important part of my life'.

Friends and relatives, too, may have been offered plenty of advice, often conflicting. Some say to them 'Never give up trying', while others say 'It's up to him, no-one else can do anything'. Sometimes the advice is 'Stick by her, even though she's making life difficult for you all', while elsewhere it's 'You must be hard; threaten divorce or she'll never do anything to help herself'. Sometimes the relatives are very embarrassed, they cover up for the drinker and try to keep their worries hidden. They may then feel alone and bewildered.

Can a problem drinker ever change?

Yes. The majority of people in trouble with their drinking change their pattern successfully or stop altogether. They usually find that life without alcohol, or with less, is not as bad as they feared, and that after some time it can be more enjoyable than their previous way of life. Often, people have stopped or cut down their drinking entirely on their own or just with the family's help. Others seek special help.

It is known how alcohol can sometimes cause harm, but at present we cannot say for certain why one person gets into difficulty while another does not. Nor can we definitely say who will recover completely from a drinking problem, and who is likely to continue drinking or to get very ill and even die.

But however small the problems surrounding the drinking, the sooner something is done the better. Once a job is lost, or health damaged or a marriage harmed, it is that much harder to put things right.

What sort of book is this?

This is a handbook: don't feel you have to read it from beginning to end. Dip into it. If you find parts helpful, underline them or mark the page. We have tried to be brief — and that means that some of the advice may perhaps sound over-simple.

When we quote former clients or patients we are using their words with their permission, direct from letters sent to us.

We would appreciate your comments on whether the book had something in it which helped you. If you feel you have tried absolutely everything here already, and to no avail, it might be worth checking if you tried consistently — because sometimes in a crisis we try anything almost at random. It will need thought to work out what is going to be best for you. In such a little book, we cannot answer all the questions you may have, but we hope you find something that helps you. *Don't forget, the odds are in your favour if you keep on trying.*

2. WHAT IS A DRINKING PROBLEM?

The effects of alcohol vary from person to person. The unpleasant effects, just as the pleasant effects — relaxation, enjoyment — depend on the person as well as the setting and the atmosphere. Alcohol makes some people noisy and jovial, others quiet and sleepy.

Having a drinking problem simply means:
- That the unpleasant side to your drinking is beginning

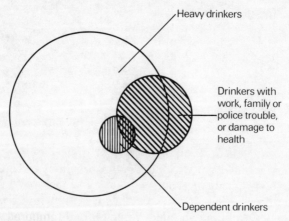

Fig. 1 Not all heavy drinkers have problems. Not all drinkers with problems are dependent on alcohol.

in some way to affect your life — your nerves, health, work, family or personal relationships; OR

● That you have become 'dependent' on alcohol, that is you are beginning really to need it, or it is becoming hard to take it or leave it [this is explained on p. 12].

You can be dependent on alcohol without having any other problems; you can also have problems, for example, in the family or at work, without being dependent.

What are the unpleasant effects on emotions and personal relationships?

Alcohol is a drug that depresses the brain. This is a fact, even though most of us know the brief, bright cheery feeling that comes with the first drink. Alcohol can actually cause severe mental depression.

Take Elaine. She had only been married a year when she suffered a miscarriage. Having been a regular drinker since 18, she turned to alcohol to dull her sense of loss. The more she drank, the more awful she felt. Yet a drink usually gave an hour or two of relaxation and release from her sadness and this was sufficient to make her continue. It was only when she stopped drinking that she realised she had recovered from her depression and was ready to go on with life. It is hard for someone who uses alcohol to dull worries and painful memories to realise it may be making them worse.

With alcohol we sometimes act very differently from normal. Although it helps us to 'let go' and this can be a good thing, for example at a party, it may also mean that the nastier side [that we all have] is more likely to come out. In some of us it brings out pettiness and jealousy towards those who are closest to us. Criticism is seen where none is intended. Drinking can make a person bad-tempered, and if alcohol brings out bottled-up envy or hate, a friendship or marriage may be threatened or destroyed.

Sometimes arguments and rows are apparently forgotten. A very high level of alcohol in the brain prevents us from remembering what we say or do. Also, the mind tends to shut out those things we are ashamed of. However, family and friends will remember.

Consider Tony. He is a civil servant, who could get quite argumentative after a few drinks. It amused him that he could sometimes wake up with no recollection of how he had got home from his club the night before. But one Sunday he was horrified on waking to discover the living room furniture scattered about, and his wife not in the house. His memory was a blank. He was afraid he had been violent to his wife. He had not, but the experience was terrifying and became a turning point in his life.

Problems in families

The person who is a regular drinker devotes time, energy and money to drinking. Sometimes this leaves the family short, not just of money, but of what he or she could be bringing to family life. Father forgets when he promises his son an outing. Mother loses interest in her teenagers. The drinking becomes a sore point. Marriages become more empty; arguments about drink take over as the chief topic of conversation — except in those families where no-one dares say anything about it for fear of causing a row. An affectionate wife turns cold and hostile, and bitter at her husband living only for the pub. A kind, considerate husband grows aloof and distant — ashamed, perhaps disgusted and insulted, by his wife's drinking. Children lose respect, becoming defiant, sulky and unhappy. They start to do poorly at school. [See chapter 8]

Problems at work

Odd days off, occasionally arriving late, or frequent sick

lines [for those hangovers and stomach upsets] are over-looked by many employers. But a day of reckoning may arise and to lose a job in this way can be demoralising. Some but not all employers want to be helpful and suspend disciplinary action if an employee with a drinking problem is determined to do something about it. After all, he is often a highly trained and valuable member of staff and it is not in the employer's interest to lose him.

The drinker often thinks no-one at work notices that for example he always drinks at lunchtime or has alcohol on his breath in the morning from last night's drinking. He may be surprised that everyone knows, long before he himself began to think he was drinking too much.

Trouble with the law

Three pints of beer, or 3 'doubles' of spirits, is sufficient to send the alcohol level in the blood over the legal limit for driving [80 milligrammes in 100 millilitres of blood]. The penalty is disqualification from driving and a fine. People who drink a lot build up a tolerance, that is they are not so obviously affected by drink. But the same amount of alcohol still gives the same blood alcohol reading.

Being publicly drunk can be an offence, especially if the person causes a nuisance. At the time of writing Britain plans to follow some other countries and provide places where drunk people can be taken to sober up instead of being taken into custody. At present, however, the usual result is an uncomfortable and undignified night in the cells and a court appearance in the morning.

In what way can alcohol damage health?

The diagram shows the ways in which moderate to heavy drinking over months or years affects the body:

7

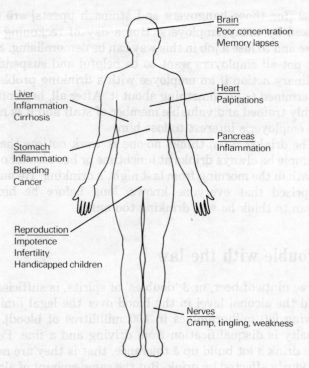

Brain
Poor concentration
Memory lapses

Heart
Palpitations

Liver
Inflammation
Cirrhosis

Pancreas
Inflammation

Stomach
Inflammation
Bleeding
Cancer

Reproduction
Impotence
Infertility
Handicapped children

Nerves
Cramp, tingling, weakness

Fig. 2 Parts of the body affected by alcohol.

The brain

Intelligence does not stop someone from becoming dependent on alcohol: authors, lawyers, doctors and professors are as vulnerable as the rest of us. However, drinking can cause a decline in intelligence and many problem drinkers cope less well on tests of thinking than they should do given their previous level of intelligence. There can even be shrinkage of the brain as the photographs show. This may be one reason why some excessive drinkers often seem at first to have difficulty making plans for the future and sticking to them. Fortunately, much of this damage to thinking ability recovers if alcohol is avoided for six months.

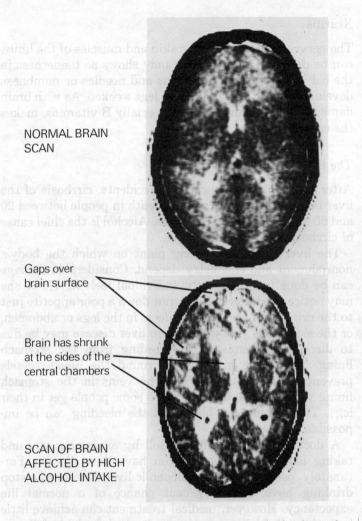

NORMAL BRAIN
SCAN

Gaps over
brain surface

Brain has shrunk
at the sides of the
central chambers

SCAN OF BRAIN
AFFECTED BY HIGH
ALCOHOL INTAKE

Fig. 3 Heavy drinking affects intelligence and can cause shrinkage of
the brain. This can happen in people who are otherwise in good health
and seem normal. The top scan shows a normal brain. The black border
is the skull bone; the shaded area is brain; the white is fluid. The lower
scan shows too much white. The brain tissue round the central fluid-
containing chambers has shrunk, and there are gaps over the surface
where shrinking has occurred.

Neuritis

The nerves that travel to the skin and muscles of the limbs can be damaged. At first this only shows as tenderness in the calves or cramp. Later, pins and needles or numbness develops and can be painful. The legs weaken. As with brain damage, lack of nourishment, especially B vitamins, makes the condition worse.

The liver

After heart disease, cancer and accidents, cirrhosis of the liver is the commonest cause of death in people between 20 and 60 in industrialised countries. Alcohol is the chief cause of cirrhosis.

The liver is the processing plant on which the body's nourishment and chemistry depend. Considerable damage can be done to it before the individual feels ill. He or she may notice tiredness and may put down a poor appetite just to the drinking. Later, fluid collects in the legs or abdomen, or the skin turns yellow. Death in liver disease may be due to disordered chemistry, or bleeding from the stomach lining. Hardening in the liver round the blood vessels prevents blood from flowing. The veins in the stomach lining swell like the varicose veins some people get in their legs. These veins can bleed and the bleeding can be impossible to stop.

A doctor is usually able to tell by examining you and taking blood tests whether you have liver disease. Fortunately, people with early alcoholic liver disease who stop drinking have a 90 per cent chance of a normal life expectancy. However, medical treatment can achieve little or nothing if drinking continues. Death invariably follows.

The digestive system

A night's heavy drinking may cause irritation of the stomach, with vomiting or bleeding. Vomited blood can be red, or brown like coffee grounds. Alcohol worsens any tendency to stomach or duodenal ulcers. In some people diarrhoea may be caused by alcohol. There is often slight damage to the intestine, which means that vitamins in food are not properly absorbed. Heavy drinkers also run short of vitamins if they don't eat proper meals.

The pancreas lies behind the stomach and makes digestive juices and insulin. It may be damaged by alcohol, causing a painful condition called pancreatitis.

Heavy drinkers are also liable to cancer in the mouth, throat and gullet.

The heart

Alcohol can cause the heart to beat irregularly or too quickly. The heart feels as if it is fluttering or gives a bumping or wobbling feeling in the chest. High blood pressure and strokes are also connected with heavy drinking.

Sex

Does alcohol increase sexual ability? Alcohol may make us feel less inhibited and apparently keener. However, in men alcohol may cause impotence. This is because a large dose of alcohol affects the nerves necessary for an erection. If this has happened once or twice a man may become worried about his sexual ability and the sure way for a man to be unable to keep an erection is to worry about it. This is what the adverts do not say: the effect of such-and-such a drink can indeed be shattering! Alcohol reduces male hormone levels, which reduces the sex drive and also reduces the chance of fathering a child.

The complexion and figure

A blotchy complexion is common in regular drinkers and, if

liver disease is developing, tiny spidery sets of blood vessels may appear on the face.

An alcoholic drink usually contains about 100 calories, but some drinkers lose weight because alcohol dulls their appetite. Those who continue to eat normally put on weight but can still be short of vitamins.

Dependence on alcohol

Some people feel they regularly need a drink at certain times or in certain situations. Some rely on alcohol believing it gets rid of tension or depression. Some depend on it to dull reality. For some, drinking has simply become such a habit that they find their routine impossible to change. These people are *psychologically dependent*. Their drinking is linked to certain triggers. Triggers may be inner emotions, such as depression or frustration, so that whenever they feel that way they find themselves thinking of a drink. Triggers can be more ordinary: passing a certain pub on the way home may set off the train of thought, or preparing the evening meal or sitting in a chair watching T.V. Ordinary

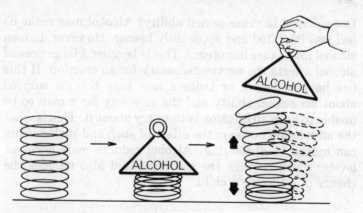

Fig. 4 Think of the nervous system as a spring. Alcohol is like a heavy weight pressing down on the spring. When the weight is removed the spring is unstable and rebounds.

habits can become very fixed when a drug is involved — and alcohol is a drug.

Alcohol is a drug which, like heroin, also causes *chemical dependence*. If alcohol is taken regularly the nervous system (the brain and its many connections) gets used to it. The nerve cells adapt. When alcohol is not there, or is there but in lower amounts, these adaptations are suddenly excessive because they are not needed. This gives a rebound effect. This rebound effect depends on how much alcohol has been drunk and for how long. Individuals vary. Five pints of beer [i.e. 5 large measures of spirits or 8-9 glasses of wine or sherry — see chart on p. 15] spread throughout the day for several months will produce chemical dependence in most people. Then the individual is out of sorts and restless for 3 or 4 days when he stops drinking.

He notices that without alcohol it is difficult to get to sleep. Even after drinking in the evening he may find himself waking at 3 or 4 a.m. — another rebound effect. In the morning he feels tense and irritable until he has a drink, perhaps at lunchtime, perhaps sooner. If dependence is severe, the tension is accompanied by sweating, trembling and nausea. These discomforts are also called withdrawal symptoms. Serious withdrawal symptoms include vomiting, fearfulness, palpitations, epileptic fits, DTs [delirium tremens]. In DTs the person loses touch with reality and sees or hears things that are not there.

The carry-over effect

People who have been chemically dependent on alcohol, and then abstain for a period, are liable to make themselves dependent on alcohol again surprisingly rapidly if they recommence drinking. It may have taken several years drinking for them to get to the point of chemical dependence, but on the second occasion the symptoms of dependence reappear much more quickly, sometimes after a week or two or even less. Even one or two days of moderate drinking are followed by the familiar and unpleasant shakiness, sickness and urge to take more alcohol. The tendency to dependence is carried over from the earlier period. Many people are affected in this way.

Is dependence on alcohol an illness?

If someone has become dependent on alcohol, there are changes in the brain cells as well as in their habitual way of reacting to life. Such people find it more difficult than the rest of us to control whether or not they drink and how much they drink. In this way dependence on alcohol can be called an illness. However, we still expect them to try to control their drinking. Their recovery will depend on how hard they try, as well as on how much help they receive.

Am I drinking too much?

If you have any of the troubles already mentioned you are drinking too much, if not all the time, at least some of the time.

But assuming all is well, you feel fine and no-one is complaining, are there any signals you should look out for?

1. Are you becoming dependent? — Are there certain situations when you always need a drink, for example, before every social engagement, or when under pressure? Is your nervous system getting so used to alcohol that 2 pints of beer or 4 drinks has no effect on you? Do you need one or two more drinks than your friends?

2. Have you tried already to limit your drinking and failed? Perhaps you simply switched to another type of drink, or you managed for a while but it crept up again? [See the Drinks Chart]

3. Have you got problems [family, money, work] which you have been ignoring or blaming on something else, but which could be due partly to your drinking or how you behave when you have been drinking?

4. A blood test from your family doctor may shown an abnormality.

5. Are you drinking to solve a problem? You may rapidly find yourself drinking too much — and end up with two problems!

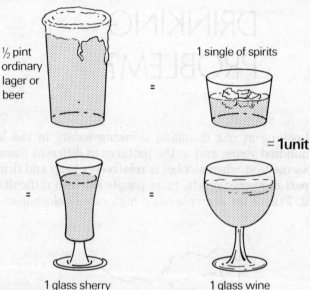

½ pint ordinary lager or beer

1 single of spirits

= **1 unit**

1 glass sherry

1 glass wine

Fig. 5 Alcohol content of various beverages. Each of the above contains the same amount of alcohol — 1 unit (8 grams).

The Drinks Chart: the alcohol content in various drinks.

Ordinary beer and lager, sweet stout:	½ pint	....	about 1 unit
Export beer, stout:	1 pint	....	about 2½ units
'Special' lager, 'diet' lager:	½ pint	....	2 units
	16 oz. can	....	3 units
Cider: (strength varies)	½ pint	....	1–2 units
Table wine:	1 bottle (75 cl)	....	8 units
Sherry, port, 'tonic wine', vermouth	1 bottle (75 cl)	....	14 units
Spirits (gin, whisky, vodka, liqueurs, Pimms, aniseed drinks such as Pernod)	1 bottle (75 cl)	....	30 units

3. CAN ANYONE DEVELOP A DRINKING PROBLEM?

Looking at our changing drinking habits in the last two hundred years, and at the patterns in different countries, it seems that when alcohol is relatively cheap and drinking is part of everyday life, more people run into difficulties with it. France for example has a high rate of alcoholism: nearly

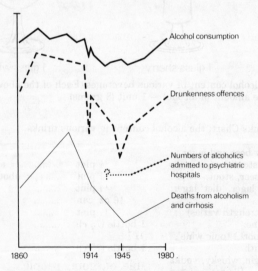

Fig. 6 The number of people with drinking problems depends on the national level of drinking.

every third hospital bed there has a patient suffering from some hazard of drinking. The graph shows how the number of people with drinking problems varies when the national level of drinking varies. However, some of us are more likely to develop a problem than others.

Does problem drinking run in families?

Yes. A man or woman whose father or mother had an alcohol problem has a high risk of following in their footsteps. As teenagers we vow we will never be like Father or Mother, but we wake up one day in adult life to discover that in some ways we are the image of them. A tense worrying nature can be handed on. We may have a tendency to cope with stress in the same way a parent did. Or perhaps what is passed from parent to child is something to do with the way alcohol affects the brain or the body.

Do some jobs put you at risk?

Drinking problems are commoner in people from certain occupations:
● Jobs where alcohol is readily available and drinking is part of the way of life [the drink trade, sales representatives, certain company directors]
● Jobs where people are away from their families [at sea, in the armed services, salesmen, the construction industry]
● Jobs where there is relatively little supervision, [lawyers, doctors, journalists].
As you might expect some of these jobs attract people who already drink regularly.

Is personality important?

It is often successful, sociable, outgoing people who turn out in their 30s and 40s to have developed a drink problem.

17

They may then become depressed, tense, suspicious or worried; but this is the result of alcohol and the trouble that has piled up. Occasionally tendencies to worrying, depression or feelings of inferiority have been there since adolescence and drinking has been an unsuccessful attempt to banish those feelings. However, people with a drink problem do not necessarily have some deeply buried twist in their personality. Once he or she has stopped drinking life becomes satisfying and productive again.

Is stress important?

People mean different things by stress. To some it conjures up the business man besieged by unfinished paperwork, unable to delegate, who does not take time out to relax. He may use alcohol to unwind at 6 p.m. without necessarily improving his temper with the family in the evening [if he gets home in time to see them].

To others stress means the bickering and nagging in an unfortunate marriage; the burden of coping unsupported with unruly children; the frustration and demoralisation of unemployment; or the worry of looking after an elderly parent.

Bereavement, particularly for the person with few relatives or friends can cause prolonged pain. Sometimes people drink to dull this pain.

All of these kinds of stress and many others can contribute to a drinking problem. However, these are difficulties which often are made gradually worse in the long run by drinking. They are sometimes difficulties which with careful reflection, and perhaps guidance, could be rapidly overcome by a change in attitude or in one's way of reacting. [More of this in Chapter 7].

Occasionally stresses are more imaginary than real. They are convenient excuses for putting off doing something about a deeply engrained habit, which has now become troublesome. People often say: 'It's my boss (or my wife) who makes me drink', when in truth it is the drinking and the behaviour that goes with it that has made the boss or the spouse critical.

Are the young immune?

Socialising and nights out almost always involve drinking so it is not surprising that many people in their teens and twenties have a spell when they are drinking a lot. Usually marriage and young children change all that! Or other interests develop or the job makes new demands. But the young person whose habits have become very set, and who begins drinking more than 3 or 4 units [p. 15] every day in addition to social outings is at risk of becoming dependent on alcohol — even if everything else in life is going well. *Specially at risk is the young person who has not found satisfaction in personal relationships or a job and who makes drinking his or her main hobby. He or she is best to be careful about alcohol and look into other ways of making life more exciting and more enjoyable.*

Can the elderly be affected?

The cost of alcohol is one reason why the over-70s appear less often in the statistics. However, the elderly do become

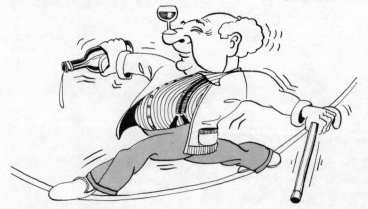

dependent on alcohol, sometimes apparently out of the blue. Depression may be the cause, or the death or disablement of husband or wife. Falls and fractures (so dangerous in the elderly) are sometimes the consequence of excessive drinking. Premature senility is another hazard. As we get older, alcohol more easily affects our intelligence as well as our balance mechanism.

4. HOW ARE WOMEN AFFECTED?

In this book we often say 'he' rather than 'she'. But with more shops and supermarkets selling alcohol, greater advertising, and changing attitudes to drinking, the number of women with a serious drink problem has increased in recent years. *Today there is nearly one woman affected for every two men.*

Serious problems from alcohol such as liver disease and physical dependence develop more quickly in women than in men, and women require less alcohol to be seriously harmed.

In those families where mother is the backbone rather than father, the effect of a mother who is emotionally unavailable because of drinking soon shows up. But much of her drinking may be hidden because she feels ashamed and guilty.

Janet, 32-year-old mother of two boys, is married to an engineer who spends two or three night per week away from home. She began to drink as a teenager 'so that she could be popular and extrovert instead of shy'. After marrying she and her husband led an active social life and both drank regularly. She began meeting her friends for bar lunches and having a vodka before her husband came in from work. She noticed she needed a drink more and more to relax and that she was easily tired. She knew she was drinking too much but felt too ashamed to speak to anyone about it. She found it very difficult to cut down. Even when she noticed her eyes becoming yellow, she could not bring herself to see her doctor. When she was finally admitted to the hospital liver unit it was a tremendous relief to be able to speak frankly to her husband and family. She decided to stop drinking completely and 4 years later has had no difficulty sticking to that. Her liver has recovered.

Alcohol and pregnancy

Women who drink heavily in pregnancy increase the chance that the baby will be small, frail, backward or even deformed. *It is harmful to the unborn child to drink during pregnancy.*

What causes a woman to drink excessively?

There are many possible influences:

● Perhaps one of her parents had a drink problem, and she never learnt to drink normally.

● Perhaps she uses alcohol to dampen tension or escape depression. She may have come to believe that she is a person of little worth. Even though the first one or two drinks still give her a temporary feeling of superconfidence, overall the drinking is probably making her feel even worse about herself.

● Perhaps she is disappointed with her marriage. If her husband devotes most of his energy to his work or hobbies she may resent carrying the burden of the children and feel her life is monotonous and unrewarding. Her husband may not have realised this or know that she feels unappreciated or needs more affection. If because of her drinking her husband has become critical of her and bossy, this will be a further hurt to her self-esteem.

● If she is an older woman she may be experiencing the loneliness of bereavement; or the emptiness of her home and life now that the children have left, especially if her husband is preoccupied with his work and she is still a housewife.

● If a woman is married to a problem drinker she sometimes begins drinking in an attempt to keep up with, or control, her husband's drinking. Women sometimes become dependent on alcohol in this way.

5. SHOULD I CHANGE MY DRINKING PATTERN?

Try making a balance sheet showing in one column the good things about your drinking and in the other column the negative things, the drawbacks of your drinking.

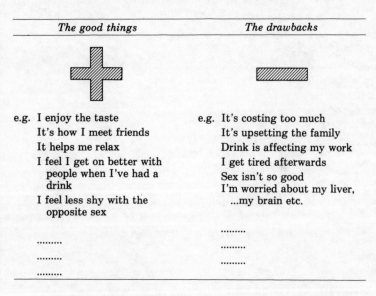

The good things	*The drawbacks*
e.g. I enjoy the taste	e.g. It's costing too much
It's how I meet friends	It's upsetting the family
It helps me relax	Drink is affecting my work
I feel I get on better with people when I've had a drink	I get tired afterwards
	Sex isn't so good
I feel less shy with the opposite sex	I'm worried about my liver, ...my brain etc.
....	....
....	....
....	....

Of course there have been, and probably still are, many good points about drinking. But a time may come when these are outweighed by the problems it causes. If the columns don't balance, a decision to do something about your drinking is logically the next step. Try to be honest, with yourself at least.

But is the drinking the real trouble?

"Drink isn't my problem, it's the answer to my problems." If a person has begun to drink in an attempt to solve a problem it can be very hard for him or her to see that alcohol has become a problem in itself. Though alcohol helps tense people to relax, regular drinking increases tension because of the frequent minor 'withdrawal effects' [p. 13]. Though alcohol may seem a stimulant it achieves this by releasing inhibitions. For a short time you may feel 'freer'. However the depressing effect lasts longer than the stimulant effect. Though enough alcohol dulls mental as well as physical pain, it does this by depressing the nervous system — and mental depression makes pain worse. These are some of the reasons why drinking to solve mental distress can actually worsen it.

Or is the real problem my job?...or my partner?...or my family?

Of course there may be difficulties with colleagues, husband, wife, parents. Alcohol, or the friendly atmosphere of the pub, provide a welcome escape but seldom an answer. Perhaps your partner/parent/employer is not going to change anyhow. Putting the blame on them is not going to improve anything.

....and who says so?

Most of us get irritated if someone makes critical comments about our habits or lifestyle. It is worse if we feel guilty or ashamed already. An angry retort from us may make the critic conveniently back off.

Sometimes, however, we need others to help us see things the way they really are. Most of us can shut out from our minds things we did that we would rather forget. Memory for what happened on drinking days is particularly liable to be patchy.

I'm at my best when drinking

Occasionally people say: 'I am someone who needs it — I'm at my best when I've had a few. It adds a new dimension to my life. Look at the poets, painters, composers who were drinkers; look at Winston Churchill'. That may be. But if you have a problem in your life, concentrate on that, not the next man. It's not very creative to make yourself ill through drinking.

I'll lose my only pleasure in life

It's a matter of weighing up the advantages against the disadvantages of your drinking. Life without your style of drinking IS possible. Lots of people have gone along the path you are now contemplating.

Should I just cut down, or stop all together?

Some problem drinkers decide to continue to drink and manage to avoid further problems. They make a radical change, not only reducing what they drink on any one occasion [e.g. never more than 2 or 3 drinks] but also cut back on how often they drink [e.g. never more than 2 or 3 times per week].

By all means try reducing rather than stopping. If it does not work, be honest and avoid looking for excuses. In our experience, and according to research findings, *abstinence is essential if any of the following apply to you*:

● If you have had symptoms of dependence for several months or more [p. 13].

● If your husband or wife is not in agreement with your plans for limited drinking [i.e. if any drinking sets up tension].

● If you tend to be someone who is easily upset, or does things very much on the spur of the moment.

● If you are not good at making rules for yourself: with abstinence there is one simple rule for every occasion — no alcohol — and that is easy for your family and friends to understand too.

● If you have damaged any of the body's organs [such as the liver] through drinking.

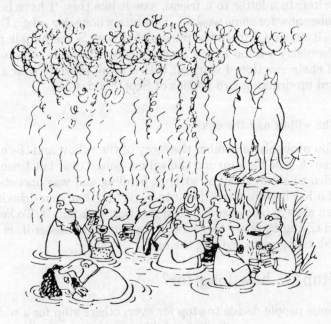

'Some people just never learn'

If you are going for cutting down rather than abstinence, read p. 39 and check the stories of Alan and Bill.

Many people find it easier and more effective to stop altogether, because they can never be sure how a drinking occasion will end. Tom is typical of a number of people with drinking problems. He writes: 'Sometimes, indeed quite often, I could and did drink without any bad reactions, but I could never be *sure* that tonight was not going to be the night when I lost control of myself. It was like playing Russian roulette with a bottle instead of a gun. Every so often I pulled the loaded chamber, and blew my brains out'.

Or you may find that although single drinking occasions never end up excessive, there is a gradual tendency for drinking to increase considerably over a few weeks — those first days when drinking is light and pleasant are the thin end of a wedge. Raymond Chandler, the detective thriller writer, in a letter to a friend, saw it like this: 'I have been sober now for some weeks — absolutely bone-dry sober. Dull as it may be, I intend to remain that way. Something in my chemistry will no longer accept alcohol. There is some sort of chain reaction. I start off with a drink of white wine and end up drinking two bottles of Scotch a day'.

The willow and the oak

You probably remember the story of the willow and the oak tree. A gale blew up and the willow bowed over but the oak tried to stand straight without bending and was uprooted. If it has become too difficult to be certain that your drinking can always be controlled then it is best to admit it. To keep on trying to prove to yourself that you can master it, is to risk being uprooted like the oak.

Stop?.....how long for?

Some people decide to stop for ever, others stop for a while and recommence limited drinking once the stresses and strains of the problem period have diminished, the brain has cleared and constructive thinking is again possible. Drinking again is safer if the new pattern is totally different from the old pattern [i.e. when, where and with whom]. But why not cross this bridge when you come to it. Leave it to next year to worry about whether to drink next year. Take a day at a time. The important thing is to have decided to do something about it.

I see all this, but it does not apply to me

Of course perhaps none of this applies to you. But because none of us like to make a critical examination of ourselves, just give this chapter a moment's reflection for two reasons:
1. To be sure you are seeing yourself as others see you.
2. To check whether your real objection is to do with a fear of losing face. [— 'No-one is going to convince me I've got a drink problem'].

Take for example Ian, a bank branch-manager who was temporarily suspended from his job. He wrote: 'The major problem is to realise that you have a problem. I knew deep down that I had; but kept saying that I had had a drink today because of some stress and that tomorrow I would not have the stress — but I still had that drink...When things got out of hand and I was forced to admit it I was ashamed. On my first visit to my doctor I told him it was a minor problem which was a lie. As soon as I was able to admit to him that the problem was a real problem the 'cure' began'.

6. HOW TO SUCCEED

Preparing for change

The big question is — do you really want to change your drinking pattern? If you really do, you will probably succeed. Making up your mind is what counts.

I've tried before but I could not stick to it

Lots of people try several times before altering their drinking. But the circumstances are never exactly the same twice. If you fear you will miss drink greatly, remember that the desire usually gets less the longer you manage without it.

If I stop drinking spirits will that be sufficient?

If your carefully considered aim is only to cut down, it may be a useful strategy to move to a dilute form of alcohol such as shandy or ordinary lager. You can make that sort of drink last longer. However, half a pint of lager contains as much alcohol as a single of spirits. And it is a fact that men and women who have drunk only ordinary beer, lager or cider have died of alcoholism. So keep an honest eye on your total intake.

Be clear about your reasons

Think through the reasons for changing your drinking habits. You might decide: 'my health will improve', or 'I'll save some money' [Why not work out how much?], or 'my family will be happier' or, 'I'll get on better at work'. Why not take a sheet of paper now and write down your own reasons?

Be clear about your decision

Try to be absolutely clear about the limits you are setting yourself. Or if you decide to stop, set a target [a month..a week..or just a day] and fix a day to check up on how it went, to reward yourself, and to set the next target. Tell your decision to a friend or someone in the family and make an agreement to let them know how you manage. Plan to save the money you don't spend and put it towards something to look forward to — a holiday for example. At present prices 6 pints of beer a day adds up to £160 per month.

Planning ahead

Don't let tricky situations catch you out. Plan in advance what you will do if you meet one of your 'triggers' [p. 12].

If time is likely to weigh heavily on you at first, think ahead to what you might do. Maybe you like reading, crosswords, listening to music or do-it-yourself? [There are suggestions on p. 36]

Do I need special help?

Yes — if you have tried several times before and failed.

Yes — if you have no-one close to check with you on your progress.

Yes — if you have had serious withdrawal symptoms in the recent past [fits, hallucinations, or severe shaking].

Yes — if you feel afraid of a future without alcohol because it has been your only escape from intolerable worries or fears.

Caution: If you are going for help merely to pacify your family, your employer or your conscience, think twice. If that is the case you probably won't be putting much into your treatment, and so you won't get much out of it. Go for yourself, because YOU WANT to do something about your drinking and your life.

Immediate survival — the first week

Will I have withdrawal symptoms?

The more you have been drinking in the past two or three weeks, the more severe the withdrawal symptoms are likely to be. Below 14 units [i.e. half a bottle of spirits or 6 pints of beer] per day these 'rebound' symptoms are unlikely to require medical observation. Above that symptoms may be severe. Individuals react differently. Symptoms are less if you cut down gradually over four or five days instead of stopping abruptly.

Restlessness, trembling and inability to sleep are worst 24 to 48 hours after the last drink and improve gradually so that physical discomfort has passed after roughly a week. If a doctor assesses that withdrawal symptoms are likely to be severe he may prescribe tranquillisers. The pills are started on the day you stop drinking, reduced gradually over 4 to 7 days and then stopped.

What should I eat and drink?

Don't miss meals — even if you are not hungry try to eat something. Your appetite will return. If your stomach is uncomfortable milk may be soothing. Vitamin shortages need to be replaced as soon as possible. Drink plenty of fruit juice, squash, sodas or water. Don't drink more than 2 cups of coffee or 4 cups of tea per day — these contain caffeine which disturbs sleep and causes nervousness.

How can I relax during this period?

Face up to it — it may be difficult. We say more about this on page 37. Meantime, here are some tips:

● Avoid stress. It may be best to take a week off work. Change your routine.

● Take relaxing warm baths.

● Listen to your favourite kind of music.

● Go for walks.

● Get busy round the house.

● Above all, do something — anything — that will distract you from the thought that you are tense or need a drink.

● Avoid negative thinking [see Chapter 7]

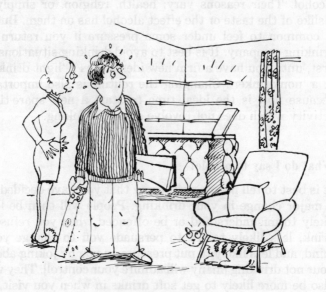

'Getting busy round the house'

Sleep

You are bound to sleep less well, so be prepared for this. But lack of sleep does not seriously harm you. Your sleep pattern will return to normal in a month or so if not sooner. It is better not to take sleeping pills, so that your normal sleep rhythm can return. Don't go to sleep in front of the T.V. Go to bed very late, read a book or paper, do a jigsaw-puzzle, and have a bedtime snack or warm milky drink.

The first few months

How do I handle parties, pubs and other drinking occasions?

Many people who regularly drink alcohol feel that if they stop they will be abnormal or outcasts. It is hard to realise at first that there are millions of people who do not touch alcohol. Their reasons vary: health, religion, or simply a dislike of the taste or the effect alcohol has on them. But it is common to feel under some pressure if you return to drinking company. It is best to avoid drinking situations at first, until you have a firm new identity as a 'light drinker' or a 'non-drinker'. Changing the routine is also important because now is the ideal time to start a new spare-time activity which does not revolve around drinking.

What do I say to people?

It is best to tell people right away that you have decided on a major change in your drinking. People will then be less likely to misunderstand or be offended when you refuse a drink, less likely to try to persuade you to change your mind, and less likely to put pressure on you by joking about your not drinking [many will admire your control]. They will also be more likely to get soft drinks in when you visit, or order you a soft drink at the bar.

Whom to tell?

You should at least tell family, close friends and drinking companions. They are likely to be understanding because they may already know there is a problem and will be relieved to talk about it.

When to tell?

As soon as possible. Putting it off makes it harder. With drinking companions try to choose a moment when they are not drinking — they are more likely to take you seriously!

What to say?

It has to sound as if you mean it. People will only take you seriously if you have obviously made your mind up. Don't let people think it's temporary — they will soon be wondering when they should start offering you your usual drink again.

For example: I've been ill recently and I've been told I'll be alright as long as I always avoid alcohol. There's something wrong with my stomach [or liver] and it reacts very badly to alcohol now, even small amounts. I've *got* to stay off it so it helps if no-one offers me a drink'. Or, 'I find one or two drinks isn't any good to me, so I don't drink at all now'.

There are bound to be occasions, socially or in the course of business, when a quick excuse is needed: 'No thanks, I'm driving'; or 'I'm on pills and alcohol is out'; or else

'I've got to keep a clear head for some desk work this afternoon'

but: *excuses wear thin, so where you can tell the truth —* '*No thanks, I don't drink*'.

What to ask for if offered a drink?

If you find a non-alcoholic drink you like, stick to it — your friends will soon know to get it for you without being asked.

Is alcohol-free lager ['Barbican', 'Danish Lite' etc.] a good choice? If cold these lagers are a refreshing non-sweet drink. But beware living out the illusion that you are still one of the beer-drinking lads — it may be time you changed that image of yourself! Do you need to make out to people that you are still drinking? Mineral waters ['Perrier' etc] with ice are fashionable, not sweet — and free of calories. Beware tonic wine, ginger wine and cider: all contain alcohol.

Suppose I still feel awkward in drinking company?

People are usually helpful if you are honest with them. Don't feel you have to apologise for not drinking. Your health and well being is what is important — don't let anyone interfere with that.

Should I keep alcohol in the house?

If you live with family or friends who drink occasionally then the atmosphere may be easier if alcoholic drinks are not removed from the house. However, if you live alone, or if your drinking was done in secret then it is wise to remove alcohol from the home.

What can I put in place of alcohol?

The answer to this depends on what function drinking has had in your life.

If drinking has been the main way of using spare time then time may weigh heavily. Avoid getting bored. Here are a few suggestions:

- Get busy round the house.

- Join the public library, not just for books but to keep in touch with the notices showing what's on in your locality.

- Take up a new hobby [you may need a few tries] — if equipment is expensive remember that you are saving money if you are drinking less.

- Take an evening class or a correspondence course.
- Make a commitment to the church or voluntary work.
- Take up a new sport; or get a pet.

If drinking has been a way of enjoying company: a new spare time activity is the best way to meet a new circle of friends. Evening classes are often friendly. Alcoholics Anonymous and the local Councils on Alcoholism [chapter 11] are ways of getting to know people in the same boat. [Loneliness is discussed on p. 46]

Get fit

You will feel better in yourself if you are physically in good condition and taking regular exercise. Take some exercise every day even if it is only walking. Local authorities offer a range of sporting facilities and keep fit classes [reduced rates for the unemployed or elderly]. Keep fit and dance classes are a way of meeting people.

Keeping it up

1. Don't let what others do or say be an excuse for drinking. *No-one but yourself is responsible for your drinking. You make the decisions.*
2. Avoid self-pity and dwelling on the past. [If you suffer from attacks of 'poor-me' read page 45.]
3. Don't be taken in. If you chose or were advised to stop and found it easy, you may catch yourself thinking you could now have the odd drink and stop again whenever you want to. Take care. There's probably a part of you that wants to get back to the old pattern again and it will produce plenty of reasons 'One won't hurt'... 'I deserve a reward'... 'It's a holiday weekend' and so on.
4. Teach yourself to relax. There are various methods: e.g. lie down or sit comfortably in a chair and systematically check each muscle in your body one by one. Start with your feet, your calves and so on up the body. To relax a

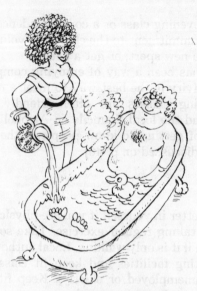

'Learn a method of relaxing'

tense muscle tighten it hard, hold it for 3 seconds, then let it go floppy and loose. Work over your whole body, finishing with your face and scalp. Your breathing should be slow and fairly deep. Sometimes simply sitting in a chair with your legs and arms resting and counting your breaths will relax you. If your mind goes on to other things, go back to counting your breaths.

5. Give yourself a reward. As Helen [p. 76] said, 'It's a good idea to spoil oneself a little. For instance, instead of buying a bottle of sherry or wine, I treated myself to a new lipstick or perfume'. You may find your savings going up quite fast if you have stopped drinking. We have often seen clients buying themselves another car or having an expensive holiday in a matter of months.

Normal drinking?

You may have decided from the start that your aim is to

train yourself to be a normal drinker. Check first on page 27 to see if you score on any of the items that make abstinence essential. Take care! This can be a recipe for disaster. If you wish to aim for normal drinking, it is vital to make firm rules for yourself such as:

● A rule about when and how much you will drink. 'Saturdays only' or 'never drink on more than two days in a row and never at lunchtimes'; 'maximum 4 units on any day [i.e. 2 pints of ordinary lager — see page 15] [6 units at a celebration]'

● Make your drinks last [sip don't gulp]; start with one or two non-alcoholic drinks.

● Buy your own drinks; avoid round buying. This is not always easy. But if you find yourself in bars sometimes, try buying your own drink as soon as you arrive before you are offered one. Or say to companions that you'll be leaving soon and so would rather just buy your own. Sometimes the others are glad not to be caught up in round buying — you probably occasionally felt that way yourself.

● Avoid drinking on an empty stomach.

● Avoid company where there is heavy drinking.

● Don't drink when depressed or angry.

● Keep a diary of your consumption to see if you are keeping to your rules.

● Be honest with yourself — get someone (a relation or a specialist) to help you see how your experiment is doing.

Here are two accounts which illustrate some of the pitfalls and possibilities:

Bill succeeded at 'normal drinking'. He had been a steady pen-pusher at head-office. He was well liked, though never the life and soul of the party. He used to go to the 'White Horse' each day after work, have two or three pints of beer and put the world to rights. Saturday and Sunday lunchtime were favourite drinking occasions when he met old friends and arranged fishing trips. Then he was promoted.

He found the new job a strain. There were too many telephone calls, too many decisions. By lunchtime he often felt tense and would unwind in the pub. By 5 p.m. he was ready for another three pints and frequently this was four to five. His wife disliked him arriving home late, intoxicated and irritable, and going straight to sleep in front of the T.V. At work in the afternoons he made mistakes and was edgy. His manager asked him to see a doctor about his nerves and his drinking. He had only once been shaky in the morning, after a New Year celebration, and had never had other withdrawal symptoms. He decided to stop drinking completely and took Antabuse [p. 76] for 8 weeks. He asked for a transfer to another department, changed his route home from work so that he did not pass his pub, and decided each Saturday to go shopping with his wife and have lunch in town. When 3 months had passed, he and his wife discussed the possibility of him drinking again. With her full agreement [though she was nervous about it at first] he began having beer on their Saturday lunch outings [2 pints maximum] and either Sunday lunchtime or evening [but not both] went to his pub for an hour before closing time for 2 pints. For a period he recorded in a diary what he had to drink. Now, 3 years later, he seldom deviates from his new pattern of drinking. He consciously avoids drinking on weekdays except on holiday. His wife is no longer worried about his drinking and he is pleased with the way things are going.

Andrew's story is different. At age 28 he took a job as a salesman. He began regularly drinking at lunchtime, and although at first this was just one or two drinks, after a year in the job it was three or four. He was away from home often and in the evening it was 7 or 8 drinks. Without alcohol in the evening he had difficulty sleeping. Without alcohol by 12 noon he was tense and and the slightest stress made him sweat. Soon he was taking a mid-morning drink, by organising his day so that he could visit a customer who would offer him a whisky, or else finish his visits early and go to a pub where he was well known. Without that his hand would tremble. One day he was charged by the police for drinking and driving. He had a discussion with his wife, and decided to stop completely. He did so for 6 weeks and then began accepting lunchtime drinks again. He soon noticed he always wanted a 5 p.m. drink if he had alcohol at lunchtime, and he always needed a 10 p.m. drink if he had been drinking at 5 p.m. Within 10 weeks his shakiness had returned. His drinking seemed to be as heavy as ever. He had another charge for drinking and driving and because it involved a serious accident he spent a night in custody. On returning home from court having had no alcohol for 24 hours he felt frightened and thought people were following him and talking about him. He was shaking all over. Tranquillisers got him through this period and he abstained for a month. But when he heard he was to lose his job he felt very sorry for himself and began drinking with his friends in the evenings. It only took a month this time for him to find he was drinking no longer for pleasure but to avoid withdrawal symptoms. He was greatly surprised at how difficult it sometimes was for him to limit his daily intake. Yet he still believed that 'this time' he would manage. Andrew had to slip a long way down, losing his job, wife and family before he was convinced that he could not be a 'social drinker'.

7. COPING WITH WORRY TENSION AND DEPRESSION

This chapter is to remind you to apply what you probably already know. Every suggestion made is simple, tried, and known to be effective. Some are comments made by people who themselves suffered with nervousness or depression and who overcame this. Here are some basic guidelines you may find helpful if you are someone who worries over the least thing, getting tensed up, so that you wish everything and everybody would go away...or that you could just get to sleep and be at peace for a few hours, or if you are someone who worries about the future, or keeps churning over past regrets so that you feel miserable and can't snap out of it.

1. **Keep busy:** If the mind is on a task, it cannot also be worrying about something else: 'the secret of being miserable is to have the leisure to bother about whether you are happy or not'.

Physical work or exercise helps. Use your muscles more and your brain less — your brain is fatigued because you are emotionally drained. Physical exercise increases the amount of the body's endorphins, substances that recent discoveries show are likely to be important in mental health.

Being with other people is another way of keeping busy — people can be your outside interest.

2. **Accept what has happened:** no good can come of regrets. Stop yourself as soon as you hear yourself saying 'If

only.....if only.....'. Brooding over regrets wastes time and valuable emotional energy. Worrying is like a rocking horse — something to do but it doesn't get you anywhere. The only point in occasionally reminding yourself of past failures or stupidity is to give yourself the strength to keep on towards your new goal.

Accepting also means not fighting what must be. If you can no longer drink alcohol safely, accept it. The ancient jujitsu masters taught that a foe could be vanquished by taking the blow and bending with it. Eventually, the foe exhausts himself. But if you struggle to resist when the odds are stacked against you, you risk exhaustion too. Many people who are not religious have found helpful the good sense in Reinhold Nieburhr's prayer [well known to members of Alcoholics Anonymous]:

> God grant me the serenity
> To accept the things I cannot change;
> The courage to change the things I can;
> And the wisdom to know the difference.

Finally, accepting means making the most of what you have. You may have lost something that you feel your happiness depended on. But you have not lost everything. Or you may feel life gave you very little. The wise man says 'what can I learn from this misfortune?... — If life gives me a lemon, then I'll make lemonade'. *It may seem over-optimistic to think a disadvantage can be turned on its head; but a crisis in life is a chance for change.* If the most is made of an opportunity for change, a new future may open up. Even if on the first attempt little progress is made, there is the satisfaction of having tried: negative thoughts are replaced by positive thoughts. *Take a risk; try something new.*

3. **Surviving failure:** things go wrong in all but the most ordered lives. 'Survivors' are people who are able to cut

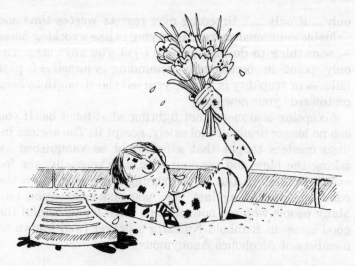

'If life gives you lemons, make lemonade!'

their losses, who get out while there is still time and shift their attention to the present and the future instead of dwelling on the past. 'This is the best I could do under the circumstances. Naturally there have been some things wrong, but it does not mean that everything I do is no good'. Two trains of thought to avoid: placing all the blame on others; or going beyond the facts and saying 'What I did was bad, therefore everything I do is bad'.

If your failures make you feel ashamed or embarrassed, take care you are not worrying about what idle gossipers are saying. Listen to what your true friends say; take the encouragement they offer.

4. Handling criticism: Dale Carnegie in *How to Stop Worrying and Start Living** [strongly recommended reading] tells how Einstein used to say he was wrong 99% of the time. So he advises: When your anger is rising because you feel you have been unjustly criticised, why not stop and

* *How to Stop Worrying and Start Living* by Dale Carnegie, Cedar Books, 1948, still in print.

44

say 'Just a minute. Einstein said he was wrong 99 per cent of the time. If that's true, maybe I am wrong at least 80 per cent of the time. Maybe I deserve this criticism. If I do, I ought to be thankful for it — perhaps I can profit by it'. The wise man is prepared to consider he may have made mistakes and learns from them.

Of course, that is the ideal. We all dislike criticism and tend to leap to the defensive: we are not cold logical beings. But a bit of cool logic can help us not to burn up with pointless resentment.

5. **Handling irritations:** let's not allow ourselves to be upset by small things, things we should scorn or forget.

6. **Self-pity is destructive:** 'People do not understand me'. 'No-one knows what I've been through'. We all have moments when this type of thinking takes over. Some of it may be pride: you may be justly proud that you have withstood so much for so long. But it can be a type of thinking that wastes mental energy. Worse, it may frighten off those who would otherwise help you. So self-pity harms you by burning up precious emotional reserves; and it harms your relationships with those around. The best cure known to mankind for a bad attack of the 'poor me's' is to think how to give another person some happiness. That may seem difficult, but think about it.

7. **Don't harbour a grudge:** bottled-up resentment eats into the soul. If you feel you have been misunderstood or shortchanged, it may be that some good can come of briefly and emphatically stating your position. You may be surprised to find that the other person is ready to admit an error. Get it off your chest — don't brood on it.

If there is nothing that can be done, then the worst mistake is to burn yourself up with the desire to get even. If it is just a matter of what the other person said or that he or she did something foolish, try reminding yourself that that person has a right to be wrong and make mistakes just as we all do. Is what he or she did so dreadful that it deserves so much of your time and energy?

8. **Someone to talk to:** People may have been saying 'It's all up to you'. As far as the drinking goes, that is 100 per cent correct — it is your responsibility. However, do not feel ashamed if you want to talk to someone about your worries. An injured leg may temporarily need a crutch and so may a stressed mind.

Obviously one should not whine and complain to everyone. Find someone you trust — a relative, friend, your doctor minister or priest. You could say something like this: 'May I talk to you? It will help me get my problem into perspective. Perhaps you can give me some advice'. Choose a moment when they will have time or arrange a special time to go back and see them. They will be pleased that you trust them.

Agencies exist where you can talk in confidence to a trained voluntary counsellor [Councils on Alcoholism — p. 79; Marriage Guidance; Samaritans; and for more practical matters, Citizen's Advice Bureau. The numbers are all in the telephone directory.]

9. **Loneliness:** People whose marriages have broken down, who have been widowed, or who for some other reason are isolated may feel loneliness acutely. It can be like a physical pain. At first a bereaved person may feel that sustaining a conversation is wearisome. They are still numbed by their loss. But at some point, as soon as possible, steps have to be taken to meet people. Meeting new people and making friends is possible for everyone, as long as you do not let yourself be discouraged if your first attempts come to nothing. Take James for example. He is a technician who lived on his own after his marriage fell apart, partly because of his drinking. He realised, too late for his marriage, that he would have to stop drinking. That was easier to bear than his feelings of loneliness. Being shy, he had never had many friends; but a colleague persuaded him to put a couple of lines in the personal columns of the local newspaper: '40-year old divorced man seeks serious friendship with woman of similar age'. No phone number just a box number

— he was so nervous that an acquaintance might find out and laugh at him. For about the cost of a round of drinks he received 30 serious replies. He contacted three of the correspondents, realising that they were just people like himself. He set out not to bore them with his own worries but to find out about them instead. He discovered that he was a good listener, which pleasantly surprised him. Far from feeling awkward, he found that if he just encouraged the other person to talk about herself, he felt completely at ease. Since he is now happily remarried he feels it was the best round he never bought.

Other ways of meeting people are more conventional: evening classes; sports clubs; church; offer your services to a local charity or voluntary organisation. For the over-65s there are lunch-clubs and pensioners' clubs [addresses from local Social Work Department]; for the widowed — CRUSE [a self-help group, to be found in the telephone directory in larger towns, which provides advice, counselling and opportunities for meeting people informally]. The personal columns of the local paper will have details of 'single clubs' and dating agencies.

10. Overcoming nervousness: The nervous system has a way of preparing us for action. When there is the need for a sudden burst of energy, for example when danger threatens, or we suddenly see the last bus about to leave, blood is diverted from the skin and abdomen to the muscles. The heart beats more strongly and faster. Muscles tighten and their balance is finely set. These reactions are useful if we are hunting dangerous animals but can be annoying, for example, for some people when they go into an interview or enter a room full of people. Most people have experienced anxiety in such situations but two factors can make anxiety into a nightmare: SELF-CONSCIOUSNESS; and THE VICIOUS CIRCLE.

The individual who is *self-conscious* thinks that the physical changes they experience when nervous, be it tremor, blushing, perspiration, are glaringly obvious to everybody and everybody who notices them is saying, 'My, that's a nervous person!'

As often as not, no-one notices anything. We know how a tiny hole in one of our teeth seems enormous to us until we actually look at it. The same applies to nervous symptoms. Other people pay little attention to them — they are interested in what we have to say and whether we appear interested in *them*.

If we get anxious because we feel the sensations of anxiety, it's a *vicious circle*. Anxiety then plagues us and we start avoiding a whole range of situations. If you are like this you should develop a relaxation method [p. 37]. Above all, as Dr Claire Weekes states in her very useful books*, do not fight it. Struggling against the symptoms can cause more tension, makes more adrenalin flow. Instead, 'float' past your symptoms. Switch into top gear and glide over them. Your anxiety will subside once you have mastered this technique. It needs practice.

Anxiety causes symptoms that may be alarming. The feeling of the heart bumping or fluttering makes some people fear heart disease. The light-headed dizzy sensation makes people fear they will pass out. This is only a fear — fainting is *very* rare in anxiety unless breathing is allowed to become excessively rapid and shallow and even then recovery is instant. A momentary blankness in our thoughts sometimes makes people fear there is something mentally wrong with them. All these fears are out of proportion. The symptoms are due to anxiety and ALWAYS pass of their own accord. Do not fight them. No-one dies of anxiety. No-one ever went crazy through anxiety.

If you are going through a bad spell with frequent anxiety even several weeks after stopping drinking, do not despair. It will pass. Accept that it may take time.

11. **Depression will pass**: think of depression as a form of fatigue — emotional draining. It always passes. The term

* *Peace from Nervous Suffering* and *Self Help for Your Nerves*' by Dr Claire Weekes, Angus & Robertson. 20 years old & still in print!

depression has a rather final ring to it. Think instead of a car engine with a flat battery. The battery needs some time, and perhaps some recharging and the engine will start again.

Very occasionally, chemical changes have taken place. If so, then the natural recovery process can be speeded up with medication [see page 76]. However, most depressions lift in a matter of days or at most a week or two.

First, do not get too worried or fearful about your state. That only makes more demands on already tired emotions. Accept. *Second*, apply what has already been said about surviving hurt, failure, criticism. *Third*, try Alfred Adler's prescription for 'curing melancholia in 14 days': 'Try to think every day how you can please someone'. Though we cannot change our emotions by deciding to, we can change our actions. When we change our actions, our feelings change too. We are less likely to feel depressed and miserable while we smile and converse pleasantly with another person. That other person can be the newspaper seller, a colleague, our neighbour, partner, or the lady next in line at the baker's shop.

12. Coping with sleeplessness: People vary in how much sleep suits them. Some people are happy with 4 hours a night, others with 7 or 8. The older you are the less sleep you need. Alcohol can make you go to sleep sooner than you might otherwise but often causes an unpleasant wakefulness at 2 or 3 a.m. This is a 'rebound' effect [p. 13]. Sleeping tablets usually do not have this rebound effect partly because the drug is still in the blood in the morning — this is why they cause a hangover in some people. Both alcohol or sleeping tablets, if taken regularly at night for a month or more, suppress the normal function of the brain's sleep centre. This gradually recovers over 3 or 4 weeks if sleeping tablets or 'nightcaps' are stopped. But during the recovery period it will at first be impossible to get off to sleep at the usual time and you dream more than usual. Eventually sleep will go back to normal.

Sleeping tablets are best avoided except for periods of less than 3 weeks and it is wise to take them on alternate nights only. Apart from long use of sleeping tablets or alcohol, the commonest cause of the feeling that sleep is poor is the belief that a magic 7 or 8 hours a night is necessary. This belief in someone who has little to look forward to in the coming day can lead to excessive worrying about sleep. Then an effort is made to get to sleep earlier and earlier, but the sleep centre cannot be willed. It has its own rhythm. The more a person worries about not sleeping the more tense he or she becomes. No-one can sleep if they are tense.

Worry is also a cause of sleeplessness. Sleep does not come if the mind is overactive and preventing the body from relaxing. At night a tired nervous system can trick you into thinking that your problems cannot be beaten. Don't be tricked. Make a list of your problems on a piece of paper and leave it till the morning when your mind is fresh. On p. 34 we made simple suggestions, such as going to bed late, relaxing in a warm bath, reading, having a bedtime snack or warm milk drink [avoid tea and coffee after 6p.m.] Physical tiredness helps so take more exercise. When you go to bed just lie still. Don't try to sleep. Remind yourself that as long as you lie still with your muscles relaxed [p. 37] you will be getting rest. If you are tense, get up and do something. Don't lie worrying. Above all do not worry about not sleeping — insomnia won't seriously harm you.

The secrets of well-being

How do people successfully come through a crisis in their lives? Successful people have not been spared set-backs, but they see these as positive experiences — opportunities for change. They rarely feel cheated or disappointed by life. They are cheerful people who have friends and who work at keeping up friendships.

They are not thin-skinned or sensitive to criticism. Survivors are people who have learnt to distinguish between the qualities and abilities of their underlying self and, on the other hand, the value they have in a given situation. Survivors do not see an attack on their work or ideas as an attack on their real value as a person, and so neither react with uncontrolled anger or defensiveness, nor absorb the blow so that it erupts later, for example, as depression or grumbling resentment.

8. HOW IS THE FAMILY AFFECTED?

When the defences go up

The family of someone with a drinking problem may suffer for years without recognition or help. The changes in the family are often gradual and at first are hard to understand. Tensions begin to build up. Perhaps the person who is drinking is erecting a defensive wall around himself. This wall is to protect himself from comment or criticism. It is also to protect the drinking which is becoming more necessary, especially if he is experiencing withdrawal symptoms when he is without alcohol. The more guilt he or she feels about the consequences of the drinking the more touchy is the response to criticism, real or merely expected. This protective wall becomes harder to penetrate. Members of the family in turn put up their own defences to avoid feeling hurt or neglected. Each person in the family becomes more isolated and the drinker becomes less and less sensitive to the real needs and attitudes of family and friends, and how they may be suffering.

Stress: uncertainty, guilt, hurt

Some of the causes of stress in the family are more obvious than others, for example, if there are financial worries or if the drinker has to face trouble at work or a court appearance.

Other stresses are less easy for outsiders to understand. There is the UNCERTAINTY and unpredictability for the family if one member has a drinking problem. Will she be alright at tea-time today, or will she be the worse for drink and bad-tempered? Will he be home on time tonight, or will I have to wait for hours not knowing when and in what state he'll return? It is very hard to plan ahead. You cannot plan meals or outings. Family life becomes highly unpredictable.

Many relatives go through a period where they feel a vague GUILT for not doing more to prevent episodes of excessive drinking. Even last resorts fail — going drinking with him in an effort to control his drinking or pouring the drink away. If you are someone who lacks confidence, the pressures when your partner, child, parent or friend has a drinking problem can reduce your confidence further. The blame for things going wrong may be laid at your door. You may even be blamed for the drinking. All manner of criticisms and accusations are hurled in moments of anger, and you may be made to feel you have failed. You may believe that outsiders blame you too.

A wife may find herself in a position where she 'cannot do the right thing'. She can begin to feel a failure as a wife, a mother and a person. She feels her only contacts with her husband are when he wants food, sex or some kind of help. Many of the HURTS are very difficult to discuss: the aggressiveness, perhaps the bed-wetting [not uncommon in people who consume very large amounts of alcohol]; the revulsion she may be beginning to feel about sexual contact.

She may feel extremely angry, but finds her angry outbursts when he has been drinking are pointless or even lead to him turning on her.

The strain of covering up

The wives of problem drinkers are often treated by their

doctor for stress symptoms — 'nerves', depression, backache, exhaustion — without revealing the real cause of their distress. The wife returns home clutching tranquillisers or a tonic because she wishes to cover up and protect her husband and herself from the shame and humiliation she imagines might come if the problem is revealed. In this way neither gets the help they really need — the agony is prolonged instead of faced. The longer the cover-up continues, the longer the drinking continues. Ask yourself if you are making the drinking *more* possible.

Practical family matters

If it is the husband who has the drinking problem, his wife sometimes has to take over some of the tasks he was responsible for — paying bills, disciplining the children, making decisions concerning the home. Drinking is expensive and in some families money cannot be found for the bills, let alone the children's school outings or new clothes. Some wives resort to taking money out of their husband's pockets at night for the next day's necessities. If it is the wife who is spending the housekeeping money on drinking the husband may find himself trying to control every penny in a desperate attempt to prevent his wife being under the influence of alcohol when the children come home from school, or he gets in from work. He ends up being responsible for the housekeeping, perhaps even stopping her getting credit at local shops — which makes her feel humiliated and angry.

How are the children affected?

Parents often say 'the children don't really know'. They are usually wrong. Even *young* children are aware if a parent has a drinking problem. Here are some of the ways children are affected:

- One of their parents is now less and less 'available' — as a guide, as a source of love, encouragement, companionship and someone they can trust.

- If their parents are getting on badly, children feel their loyalties divided. Strife between parents causes great distress to children. Older children may try to intervene; younger children withdraw. In such families, the children tend to develop problems — delinquency, aggressiveness [perhaps imitating what he has seen at home]; nervousness and fearfulness; bedwetting; physical complaints perhaps without any medical basis. The general unhappiness and stress shows up at school too, for example, falling behind in class or truancy.

- Children learn by example and are at risk of developing a similar problem later in life [p. 17]

- When a parent's drinking problem has become severe and the other parent is not coping, one of the children may find adult responsibilities thrust on him — mothers sometimes say 'he took his father's place'. Some children find the responsibilities too much, others cope well. Take John for example... John, the youngest of three sons, on the surface seemed to be perfectly stable. He was 14 when his schoolteachers asked the family doctor why John's attendance at school was so poor. His mother was drinking heavily. This always worsened her tendency to depression and her back pain from her slipped disc. She would lie in bed, feeling very sorry for herself. Her husband worked long shifts — 7a.m. to 7p.m. John felt he had to stay at home to make sure she was alright. He feared she would become intoxicated and fall; or, as once happened, go to sleep with a cigarette in her hand and burn the bedclothes. He was afraid that if he was at school she would drink more. He lost touch with his friends, stopped going to his clubs and fell behind in class. Outwardly he was the model son. Underneath he felt very resentful. When he was 16 he suddenly and angrily broke off all contact with his parents to go and live with his brother 200 miles away. His mother was deeply hurt at his complete rejection. Then, patiently she allowed time to pass for him to gain his sense of independence, and to let him and the rest of the family see that she was at last determined to tackle her alcohol problem. But during the two years that elapsed she frequently felt that she had lost him for ever.

Separation and divorce

Divorce is equally common in families where the wife has the problem, rather than the husband. Some men have real fears about the care of the children if their wife's drinking has affected day to day living and made her unreliable. Of course, separation or divorce is usually very upsetting for all the family. We know couples where in the end it turned out to be a good solution for all concerned but we know many more who worked at their marriage and did well.

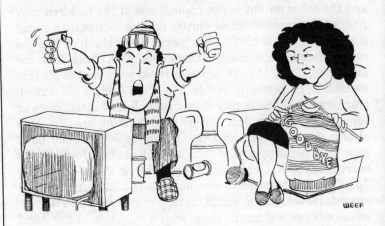

9. HOW CAN I HELP HIM?

1. First, if you want to help, let the person know that you are prepared to help and to give support if he or she is ready to make changes. Be prepared to go for help with him. Assure him that while you may feel bitter and resentful, you still care about what happens to him.

2. Let your relative know what you can and can't tolerate. But don't make him/her out to be the 'baddie' and you the 'goodie'. We all have our faults. Let your partner know if you have been feeling miserable, low, lonely, without making it seem like a further attack on him. Be ready to give appreciation and encouragement, and recognise how rarely you have been doing that lately. Be prepared to look at what you do that makes things worse and to accept criticism.

3. Be prepared to seek outside support for yourself. It may help you to understand the problem better, and to be more effective in bringing about changes. It may be hard to do it alone. Many people really do understand, many have gone through similar difficulties themselves. People care about what happens to you too. Try a meeting of Al-Anon [p. 79]. Be prepared to attend a number of meetings; give it a chance — there are no instant solutions. Or talk to someone at a Council on Alcoholism [p. 79].

4. Avoid protecting him from the consequences of his

57

drinking since that makes it easy for him to continue. Don't make excuses for him anymore.

5. Recognise that months or years of bitterness and resentment will have left some mark. You will have to put real effort into building a new life together. How much better than putting so much energy into the 'big cover-up'.

6. Don't waste energy trying to control the person's drinking. If he or she is determined to drink there is little another person can do until he or she has a change of mind. You are not responsible for another person's drinking. It is the other person who decides to take that drink. Of course, there may be times when this rule is difficult to put into practice — if you can see a particular situation coming up when to drink would have serious consequences. But it is an important principle which has helped many to free themselves from a frustrating and fruitless struggle.

How can I cope with the denial?

Your relative may minimise the drinking and the problems, perhaps even tell lies. Most of us prefer not to be reminded of foolish or hurtful mistakes. But for someone with a drinking problem to talk of giving up or reducing drinking may be upsetting in itself — alcohol, or the pub, has become a very important part of life, perhaps even a crutch. He or she may have been using alcohol to dull awareness of worries or other problems.

Confronting this denial needs the right timing. Never try when he or she has been drinking or is still intoxicated. The 'morning after' may be a good time; or if there is a crisis. Do not always try to keep the peace on the morning after. If that morning he or she is not drinking and feels wretched or remorseful, use the opportunity to explain the harm that surrounds the drinking, without it seeming as an attack. Help him to weigh up the pros and cons of his drinking and try to persuade him to make a firm decision and perhaps to

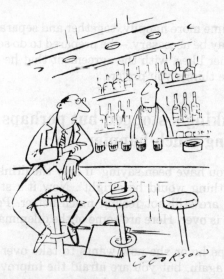

'This one's to help me unwind from the office ... this one's to help me wind up to face the wife and kids ... this one's to help me unwind after' again.

seek outside help. If he agrees to seek outside help make the appointment straight away. *Go with him.*

Don't make idle threats. Only make threats if you really mean what you say. Sometimes if a crisis is allowed to occur it may bring about important changes for the better, though it may be distressing at the time.

Though difficult, it may be useful to have a family get-together at a time when your partner has not been drinking. The childrens' understanding, caring and honesty about how they feel can be a helpful eye-opener. No parent wants his children to be unhappy and hurt by his actions. The drinker may feel the children have turned against him. They may rarely get a chance to let their father know that they care greatly about him. Never try to turn the children against your partner. Children need the love of both parents. Children should stay out of their parents' quarrels.

Try to think of the good and positive things you can all aim for. Think of different ways that you and your partner can spend time more happily, together and separately. Compromises may be necessary — be prepared to do some things that the other likes, with the agreement that he or she will join in some things you prefer.

The drinking's stopped but perhaps you're not feeling much happier

For years you have been saying 'if only the drinking would stop, everything would be alright'. Now it's stopped but maybe you are still not feeling much better. Perhaps the honeymoon is over. Here are some of the dilemmas you may face:

● Perhaps he or she now wants to take over managing the money again, but you are afraid the improvement will not last. It's hard to trust again.

● Perhaps he wants to take over disciplining the children again. You may disagree about how this should be done and the children may rebel against it. An older child will find it hard to let go of the freedom, or the special closeness with you, that he has had recently.

● Perhaps you resent the encouragement going to your partner for stopping drinking while no-one seems to appreciate all you have had to put up with and the changes you have had to make. It can be puzzling and distressing to feel this way when everyone expects you to be grateful.

● Perhaps memories are still painful. In a marriage where one partner has had a drinking problem, the other partner often takes a long time to forgive and forget especially if past injuries have left deep wounds.

Alec and Mary, a couple in their 30s, experienced some of these difficulties. Things went well for three or four weeks as Alec determined to do something about his drinking. But Mary's anger at all the broken promises of that last year was only just below the surface. She criticised his wallpapering when at last he got round to redecorating the lounge.

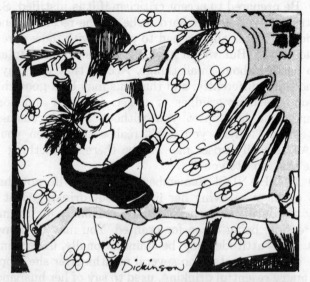

She complained when he brought the boys home late after taking them [the first time in years] to a football match. Inside she felt bad for getting angry with him when he was doing all that was asked of him. She was puzzled that she felt annoyed when their relatives gave Alec pats on the back for doing so well. 'If only they knew how hard it's been for me', she used to say to herself. Alec did not understand her grumpiness...and nearly reacted by drinking again.

Some wives are baffled at having given their husband the first drink again. They found it impossible to tolerate the atmosphere when he was sober.'He was getting on my nerves, always watching me; always restless. I went out and bought him some beer so that he'd leave me in peace'. A wife may feel inadequate when her now competent husband is around more and is now criticising HER. Perhaps your self-confidence needs building up again. Think of something you can do that will give you a sense of achievement. Your husband will enjoy having a happier and more confident wife. Ask for his support in a nice way, not in a crochety grudging way. He may be pleased to be asked.

• Be prepared to accept criticism if it is justified. Some partners have found it hard to be on the receiving end of criticism: 'After all I've had to put up with, how dare she criticise me!' But we all have our faults. Try not to enter into battles about small things. Accept that you may see some thing differently, and that this may be a good thing.

Don't harbour grudges or anger. Be open and honest about what has upset you without being accusing or attacking: "Maybe you don't realise that when you do THAT it really upset me. Maybe there's something I've done that upsets you?"

• HUSBANDS! Remember that your wife now has a new problem — living her life without drinking. But she may also still have to face some old ones: for example, depression; being taken for granted. You may be unaware that your attitude may be unintentionally undermining. One of our patients even several months after she stopped her angry resentful drinking, used to say of her husband, 'I wish I were his secretary, not his wife. I'm sure he doesn't criticise his secretary as much as he does me. I never seem able to do anything right'.

• Don't forget Al-Anon meetings [p. 79]. Al-Anon has a wealth of experience, understanding and unsentimental advice and helps families develop a more positive attitude to everyday life.

Our next chapter touches on some of the commoner problems in marriage. Some aspects of your relationship may need working on if there are to be real improvements when your partner stops drinking.

A word to teenagers

Life in the family has probably been far from easy for you lately. However if your parent has decided to begin to do something about his or her drinking problem, you may like some hints about how you can help.

Try to avoid power struggles with your parents. If you

tackle them in a reasonable way and not in a grumpy, accusing way they are more likely to be fair in return. If it's an argument about what time you are to come home, explain what you want to do. Obviously, a friendly attitude will get the best results. An affectionate hug of reassurance — he or she may feel very guilty for letting you down in recent months — may be shrugged off with embarrassment but will be greatly appreciated.

Your parent has been suffering and struggling with a problem that may take a great deal of courage and determination to conquer. You should never feel to blame for the drinking, but your care and concern shown in a loving way will be a great help.

Coping with setbacks

So your partner promised to abstain or greatly reduce the drinking. Be prepared for occasional relapses when drinking may be excessive. Take a positive attitude. Don't be too ready to accuse, but don't pretend it is not happening until it really gets out of hand. Confront your wife in a direct but caring way, and when she's NOT had a drink. Let her know you still want to work towards improving matters. Let your husband/your son know his drinking or increased drinking is affecting the family. Let him know you are still concerned for him. Set your limits, but try not to make him feel too bad or he may take refuge in more alcohol. He'll probably be feeling pretty bad already about letting himself and the family down.

Sometimes people have said that they found themselves taking a drink, and knowing there would be such anger on

$1 \times$ 🍷 *need not =* +

their return home decided they might as well have a real session and 'be hung for a sheep as for a lamb.'

If your relative starts drinking again it may be time to seek outside help. If you have already been having outside help you may fear that you will be turned away this time because things have failed. Don't let that fear put you off renewing contact. Something positive can come out of a relapse — a new understanding of what the real difficulties are. But don't spend too much effort tracing events back if he or she genuinely cannot understand why or how the relapse happened.

Don't say 'It's a disaster, we're back to square one'. Instead remind her how well she's done, and what has been achieved so far. You may be angry and disappointed, but don't lose sight of how difficult it may have been for her. Check within yourself that you, too, have not given up making the extra effort. It's easy to fall back into old habits. Positive encouragement will lead to more rewarding results than angry carping.

10. MARRIAGE AND THE SEXUAL RELATIONSHIP

All marriages go through bad patches. In some it is a matter of days, in others weeks may pass before an atmosphere of anger or resentment clears. If nothing is done to work out what is going wrong, grumpiness and tension will soon be back. If you cannot work it out it may be worth contacting a marriage counsellor. In this chapter we touch on a few of the commoner difficulties.

Communication

If you are feeling depressed, resentful or dominated because you are not getting what you want from your marriage, ask yourself 'Does my partner know what I want?' Or have you just assumed he/she does? Also ask 'What am I really giving my partner?' Is the giving one-sided or balanced?

Take Dorothy for example. When she came for marriage counselling, she used to stare at the nearest planet and say things like: 'Some people go on holidays....' Her expression varied between martyrdom and sarcasm. What she should have said was 'I'd like to go on holiday. Can we discuss whether it will be possible'. Don't assume. Be clear and frank. *It is definitely possible to be frank in a kind way, without being accusing or blaming.*

Mutual respect is important. If you feel the balance is un-

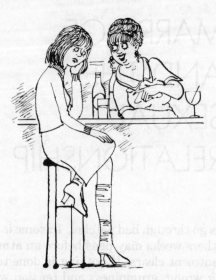

'Another marriage on the rocks, dear?'

fair or you are being taken advantage of, but are too timid to ask for what you want, then remember: no-one respects a doormat.

The other side of this coin is that we have to *listen carefully* to what our partners want because they may have difficulty putting it clearly. You can be sure however that they give clues all the time. They may often want you to be a loyal friend, a source of appreciation, encouragement or comfort.

Be a good listener. It may sometimes be difficult to change how your partner is feeling; but you will find it helps if you listen to how he or she feels. This means not immediately trying to argue or jolly them out of it, nor jumping to your own defence. *Listen!*

Giving to get

If you want changes, try to reach an agreement on what you can both do towards an improvement. Keep it simple. If it's your untidiness that annoys your husband, and one of the things that upsets you is his refusal to give you time away from the children, then sign a contract [make a bit of a joke about it] stating that you agree to keep your clothes and the kitchen tidy if he agrees to take the children out on Saturday afternoons. Run the contract for two weeks — or until one of you breaks it!. What worked for two weeks could become the pattern.

Stating the positives

When your partner makes an effort or does something kind or helpful, seize it as a chance to say something positive — thanks, appreciation or praise. Even if you do not feel warmly deep down, saying it may help you feel less cross. And it will increase the chance that your partner will make the same effort again.

Jealousy

This is a common emotion in marriages where there is a drink problem. If the jealousy is in the drinker, it may be an effect of alcohol and jealous ruminations may disappear when the drinking stops. If not, then you may need to seek advice. Or, try thinking of it this way. If you fear that someone is forcing you out, it probably means that you haven't much confidence in yourself. If you felt confident that you were desirable, capable and strong it would never occur to you to fear that you were losing your lover, unpleasant though that might be. Feelings of inferiority have to be seen for what they are: just fears in your mind. It may be high time that those fears were checked against reality. Start by making a list of your real qualities and all the things you do well. Also, recommence doing some of the things you did well in the past. *Make the most of yourself.*

Sex and your marriage

On page 11 the effects of alochol on sex were mentioned. However, frequently it is not just the drinker who is affected, but also the partner. The tension and resentments that may have built up are a powerful dampener of a sexual relationship. In a marriage where the husband being drunk disgusted his wife, she may develop a dislike even of being touched by him. He must try to understand how this came about and approach with tenderness and patience if at first she cannot respond in the way he would wish.

Bob and Jenny are typical of the many couples who reach their forties before they really try to have a more fulfilled sexual relationship. One of the chief problems was that Jenny had brought to the marriage attitudes to sex that came from a family where sex was taboo. Because it felt shameful, she had never allowed sex to be thoroughly pleasurable. It took some help from a marriage counsellor until she could accept that she was holding herself back.

Although the drinking is no longer a problem and the rela-

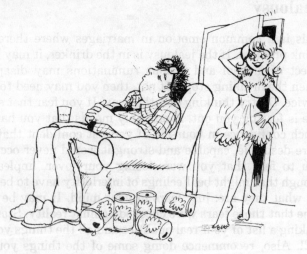

'The effect can be shattering'

tionship becomes more affectionate, there may still be tension in bed. Perhaps as in Bob and Jenny's marriage the difficulties were there before the drinking problem. Here are some suggestions which have helped many couples:

Hints

First, each should help the other to be really relaxed. Atmosphere is important! [People who have used alcohol to relax should know that in larger quantities it interferes with the male and the female body's ability to respond because of its effect on nerve fibres.] There are no rights or wrongs in sex. What is right is what gives you pleasure and what you can do for your partner that gives him or her pleasure. Tell your partner if there are ways of touching you find off-putting. Then take it in turns to show each other what you find pleasurable, by guiding the hand for example. Don't over-emphasise intercourse. Sex therapists usually ban intercourse until the couple have made new discoveries in touching and caressing, including bringing each other to a climax without intercourse. Only when both partners feel ready should intercourse happen and then only arising out of the initial pleasurable giving and getting. Experienced lovers often devote 20, 30 minutes or longer to exciting and caressing each other before intercourse begins.

Second, never worry over performance. You cannot relax and become sexually aroused if, instead of enjoying the sensations of touching each other, you are worrying about how you are performing. This is the commonest reason for a man to be impotent i.e. have difficulty keeping an erection. Again, an important step in treating impotence is for the sex therapist to ban intercourse while the couple practise touching and caressing for mutual enjoyment. *If a couple stop worrying about intercourse, they can start enjoying sex again.*

Some women who have drinking problems have used alcohol to dull the mind and make sex tolerable because they feel guilty or frightened about sex. If such tension persists despite a loving relationship and tender love-play then go for help. Dr Devlin's *Book of Love** is well worth reading. Read it together! But if you have a problem that is persisting why not ask your doctor about it? If he cannot help you ask him to refer you to a specialist, or make enquiries yourself. Family Planning Clinics and Marriage Guidance Councils often provide sex therapy or can redirect you.

Working at marriage*

Any marriage has to be worked at. It cannot be expected simply to run itself. One kind of effort that is needed is the effort it takes to forgive and accept. If your partner makes a blunder, how much pleasanter it is for him or her if the damage is quickly repaired and the long lecture by you is missed out. The same applies to those annoying habits he or she has. If they cannot be changed, don't go on making mountains out of molehills. None of us is perfect. Accept your partner's irritating habits and failings just as you want most of yours accepted. And why not list his or her virtues for a change?

---

* *The Book of Love* by Dr David Devlin, New English Library, 1974, about £1.75

* For an unsentimental account of marriage problems and how to tackle them read *Making Marriage Work* by Paul Hauck, Sheldon Press, 1979, about £1.95

11. CAN FRIENDS OR COLLEAGUES HELP?

Typically friends, colleagues and supervisors at work try to shield the individual with a drinking problem. For example, they take responsibility for jobs that have not been done, or make excuses to the management. Perhaps they say to themselves, 'I'd drink myself if I had to put up with her mother-in-law/his loneliness/his strain at work'.

Friends, supervisors, employers or colleagues who cover up for the drinker, or ignore the signs, are often harming him or her, not helping. As long as a crisis or confrontation is avoided, the person can continue to drink and harm may result. The crisis which everyone seems so intent on preventing — in the work setting, disciplinary action for example — could actually be a turning point. Sympathy on its own may change nothing, whereas intervening promptly and perhaps pushing the individual into doing something constructive may prevent the problem developing.

Having an honest open discussion in these circumstances may not be easy. If the individual is on the defensive, he may try to make you feel a 'drag', a spoil sport: 'Come off it! What's wrong with a drink or two? You're a wet blanket these days!' Or, if you are the employer or manager he may even accuse you of victimising him. You can say, however, that it is not your business to diagnose a drink problem: you want an improvement in your friendship — or an improvement in work performance — and that you want him to seek specialist advice. As employer you may wish to add that he should agree to follow whatever treatment is recommended. The National Councils on Alcoholism [p. 83] offer information about policies that organisations can follow. If you are just a friend, you will find much of the advice in Chapter 8 applies to you and you are also welcome to attend meetings of Al-Anon (p. 79).

12. GOING FOR ADVICE

Medical and psychiatric help

Your family doctor will understand the problems that arise from excessive drinking and can advise you *if you put him fully in the picture*. He will not necessarily send you to a specialist, but may do so if asked, or if he feels it will be helpful. He may prescribe vitamins, deterrent drugs ['Antabuse' or 'Abstem'], or tranquillisers for 4 or 5 days if serious withdrawal symptoms are likely.

Psychiatrists are doctors who have had special training in mental illness and also, perhaps, drinking and drug problems. Psychiatrists seldom ask you to lie on a couch, hypnotise you or give electric shocks. Nor do they have a magic wand. If you are referred to a psychiatrist he may simply offer you and the family doctor some advice. Or he may see you for a series of appointments during which he may go into your background and your present life in order to help you see more clearly what will need to change in order for you to cope more successfully. Don't expect a psychiatrist to hand you a bunch of excuses for your drinking. Perhaps you were unfortunate enough to have had a miserable childhood — but today you are the only one responsible for your drinking.

For many people stopping drinking or cutting down is the

73

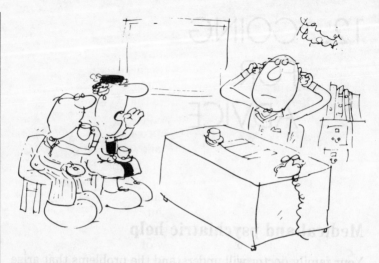

'I said, "And that's another thing I can't stand — the way he slurps his tea"'

solution to their difficulties. Occasionally after a honeymoon period some of the old personal problems rear their heads — shyness, feelings of inadequacy, resentments, sexual difficulties. A psychiatrist or psychologist may be able to help at this point. *But there is no miracle cure to any of these problems and the therapist will expect you to work patiently at changing your attitudes and beliefs.*

Tests a doctor may do

Drinking affects the liver and the blood cells. Simple blood tests that your general practitioner can do will show the extent of this.

What if I want to see a psychiatrist?

To see a psychiatrist either though the NHS or privately it is usual to ask your family doctor to refer you.

Special clinics

The staff in specialised centres may be doctors, nurses, psychologists, social workers or specially trained lay people who are sometimes recovered problem drinkers. In general today these clinics do not assume that everyone who comes is an alcoholic who must never drink again. Most clinics include group discussions in the programme. The group will consist of one or more staff and other patients whose problems are likely to have some element in common with your own. It helps overcome shame and secrecy to meet others with whom you can identify. As experiences are shared your own difficulties fall into perspective. You begin to see things as others see them [while drinking you may have had a rather one-sided view of events]. Not all groups are just for discussion — for example, instead of theorising about how to refuse drinks at a party the group might actually practise doing it.

Do not be surprised if the clinic wants to contact the family. It is important to have the family's views. Also the clinic may have useful information and advice for them.

All this may be as an out-patient or an in-patient. Admission makes the treatment a more intense experience, but is seldom absolutely necessary. People tend to be admitted if withdrawal symptoms are likely to be severe; or if stopping drinking or cutting down has proved impossible while living at home; or if the staff feel there is some important side to your problems that needs closer attention.

Two-thirds of people who go to special clinics are greatly improved a year later.

Can I contact a special clinic myself?

Some centres welcome enquiries and will offer appointments direct; others prefer their clients to be referred by a family doctor.

Medication

Tranquillisers

These can lead to addiction if taken over a long period — they become less effective and a need is felt to build up the dose. Then withdrawal symptoms begin and a vicious circle is set up. Therefore they are best used only for a few days at a time, for example, in the 4 or 5 days after stopping very heavy drinking. Sleeping tablets should also only be used for very short periods, if at all [see p. 49].

Antidepressants

A small number of people who are depressed, usually those whose depression is severe and fits the medical syndrome of 'depressive illness', benefit from these drugs. Antidepressants correct chemical imbalances in the parts of the brain that control mood. Those in common use are not addictive, are safe, and if you are advised to take them the prescription should be followed closely.

Deterrent medication

'Abstem' and 'Antabuse' are substances which if taken regularly in the correct dose cause an unpleasant, even dangerous, reaction if alcohol enters the body [flushing, headache, nausea, pounding feelings or faintness]. If the aim is to stop drinking completely, these pills are a useful insurance policy. Once you are taking these pills you know that you must not drink for at least 5 days [7 in the case of Antabuse].

Helen's husband was a busy company director, a reserved man at the best of times, and she often felt he ignored her, even belittled her. A pattern of drinking developed whereby she often was drunk when he arrived home. She knew she was driving him further away; she felt disgusted with herself. Yet only two or three weeks later once more she would find herself feeling hurt about something, buy a bottle of sherry and escape into semi-consciousness again. As tension mounted in the marriage she felt more and more depressed till during one drinking session she tried to kill herself. At that point, realising that she could not expect her husband to change overnight into someone always warm and caring, she decided to take Abstem. She wrote to us: 'Being on Abstem was the most tremendous help. Having to be without the crutch of alcohol meant I was able gradually to build up confidence in myself and come to realise that I could do everything I wanted to and do it well'. She found a part time job and this time kept it, took a class at college, and worked at being more independent and confident.

For the person who *wants* to abstain, these medicines help establish a period of stability in which to get life reorganised. Injured self-esteem has a chance to recover. Determination has time to become established. It gives a chance to find out that life without alcohol is possible.

Is it weakness to rely on a pill instead of willpower?

The trouble with willpower is that it is not always at its best when you need it. With these pills a decision to drink or not to drink still has to be made, but only once a day.

Is there anything I should avoid?

When taking these pills avoid food that contains alcohol such as some trifles; large quantities of vinegars made from wine or cider or pickles using such vinegar; after shave, hair tonic; alcohol-based back rubs; eau de cologne; cough medicines that your chemist says contain alcohol. If, when out, you are afraid 'friends' may spike your drink, keep your eye on it.]

Vitamins

Heavy drinkers often run short of vitamins, especially B

vitamins. These can be bought at chemists or health food shops or obtained on prescription. Vitamin injections are sometimes necessary.

Alcoholics Anonymous

Much of the present-day concern and sympathy for the problem drinker is due to A.A., whose members for 40 years have shown the world that a man or woman can have a severe drink problem but may want to recover and can achieve this. A.A. has grown spectacularly in the past 10 years. It exists only to help individuals overcome the problem. There are no membership fees. The only requirement for A.A. membership is a desire to stop drinking. At an A.A. meeting there is a warm informal welcome for newcomers — it is a fellowship in which all have in common the fact that their drinking at one time or another caused harm. During the meeting, members talk about their own experiences. The newcomer learns that others have had similar experiences with alcohol. He learns that he is not alone. Most important he learns that recovery is possible.

'What's the point', some people say, 'of going over your own story again and again?'. Paul explained as follows: 'To remember just how bad my life was when I was drinking is important to me today. I was a very sick person when I finally reached out for help. I had lost the will to go on living. I was utterly beaten. I don't want to forget where I came from. If at a meeting I can pass on the tiny ray of hope that was given to me and changed my life three years ago then I am truly grateful for the opportunity to be able to do so'.

A.A. members have not found it possible to drink again with any certainty that it will be safe. They recommend abstinence. They know the relief that comes when the problem drinker ceases to struggle to control his drinking, admits he has lost the fight and surrenders to the realisation that he is 'powerless over alcohol'.

Some A.A. writing and speaking is spiritual. People whose lives have been transformed since starting to go to A.A. feel that there must have been a guiding force helping them to achieve what they have achieved. Who knows? It is possible. But do not be put off if you are not a religious person and a member mentions God. Just as with any approach, take out of it what you need. There is wisdom stored up in the customs and sayings of A.A., and a vast understanding of people who drink. Give yourself 3 or 4 meetings to allow you time to begin to see how it works. In most areas there is more than one meeting — try several.

How can I contact A.A.?

Look in your local newspaper, phone directory or directory enquiries under Alcoholics Anonymous. Your Citizen's advice bureau may also give a number to call or tell you the time and place of a meeting in your area. [see Appendix]

Al-Anon and Al-Ateen

Like A.A., Al-Anon groups can be found in most cities and large towns in Britain. The members are husbands, wives, parents, children and friends of people with drinking problems. They offer advice and support.

Al-Anon is not the place for people to moan about what terrible husbands they have. People are there to talk about where they may have gone wrong without being made to feel guilty, and to work out how they can take a more effective attitude to their problems. The approach is warm, welcoming and above all understanding. Go to several meetings before deciding whether or not their approach will be useful to you.

How can I contact Al-Anon?

Via Alcoholics Anonymous, or see Appendix.

Councils on alcoholism; advice centres

Councils on Alocholism are voluntary bodies, usually with one or two paid staff. They offer advice, information and sometimes counselling. No charge is made to clients though donations are accepted. They have strict rules about confidentiality. There is sometimes an informal social side to their activities which is helpful to the person who is having difficulty making new friends or spending his spare time.

How can I contact them?

Phone for an appointment or just go along. Check local phone book or newspaper or obtain the address of your nearest Council from the National Office [see Appendix].

Residential help/hostels

Isolation is common among problem drinkers who have lost touch with family and friends. Many cities have living-in facilities for such people, if they are in the process of trying to find a new lifestyle. These are run by social work departments, voluntary organisations or one of the churches. Skilled help is available, but residents are usually expected to take an active part in the running of the hostel. Abstinence is usually the goal of residents. Although you may have your own room, the emphasis is on living as a member of a group. These facilities are not to be confused with lodging houses or shelters for the homeless.

How do I contact them?

Through your local social work department or Council on Alcoholism.

Other organisations

See Appendix.

13. SURELY IT'S NOT THAT EASY?

For many people, once they have made a decision to do something about their drinking, it is easy. Others may have a number of false starts. For them it becomes a matter of experimenting to find the best strategy — but scientific experimentation requires an honest objective unbiased observer so if you are having repeated experiments you should seek help from an outsider.

If trying to become a normal drinker is not working out, you should have a period of several months completely free of alcohol.

If you have set out to abstain but find you keep 'breaking out', EITHER:

● Plan an attempt at normal drinking, closely following the guide on page 39, and with a third party to give you honest advice about it. OR

● Contact A.A.; or request a deterrent drug for a period from your doctor; or get an appointment at a special centre.

Ian [p. 29] who chose abstinence as his best solution put it like this: 'I assure you it's not all fight. In fact, I must say that it was easier than I imagined. At the beginning, one reason why I had not wanted to admit my problem was that I imagined giving up would be so difficult. I am not saying stopping drinking was easy, but with an understanding wife, some professional help and a wish to succeed, it was easier than I had feared...Now I see that the fact that I drank, that I felt I needed it and could not do without it, was a state of mind. Now I've changed my way of thinking. I've re-programmed myself'.

Never give up trying to find your solution. The odds are in your favour.

APPENDIX: ADDRESSES OF AGENCIES OFFERING HELP

Councils on alcoholism

These are to be found throughout the United Kingdom. The address of the Council in your area can be obtained from one of the following:

Alcohol Concern, 3 Grosvenor Crescent, London SW1X 7EE. Tel 01 235 4182

Scottish Council on Alcoholism, 147 Blythswood St, Glasgow G2 4EN. Tel 041 333 9677

Northern Ireland Council on Alcoholism, 16 College St, Belfast BT1 6BX. Tel 0232 238173

Irish Council on Alcoholism, 19/20 Fleet St. Dublin 2. Tel Dublin 774649

Alcoholics Anonymous

There are about 1000 groups throughout the U.K. and Eire. Information from:

Alcoholics Anonymous — U.K. General Services Office, P.O. Box 514, 11 Redcliffe Gardens, London, S.W. 10. Tel. 01 352 9779.

Scotland: 50 Wellington St. Glasgow Tel. 041 221 9027.

Northern Ireland: Central Service Office, 73 Lisburn Rd, Belfast 9. Tel. 0232 23305.

Eire: Service Office, 26 Essex Quay, Dublin Tel. Dublin
774809.

Al-Anon

Al-Anon Family Groups U.K., 61 Dover St., London SE1
4YF, Tel. 01 403 0888.

Voluntary Organisations

ACCEPT has several centres in and near London: contact
ACCEPT, Western Clinic, Seagrave Rd, London SW6 1RZ.
Tel. 01 381 3155.
LIBRA: 19 Landsdown Place, Lewes, Sussex BN7 2JU. Tel.
07916 77100.
DRINKWATCHERS: c/o ACCEPT [see above].

FURTHER READING

Books and pamphlets on recovering from alcoholism, and advice for the family may be obtained by post from Alcoholics Anonymous — U.K. General Services Office [see above] and from Broadway Lodge, Old Mixon Rd., Weston-Super-Mare, Avon, BG24 9NN. Tel. 0934 812319.

Alcoholism by Dr Max Glatt. Teach Yourself Books, 1982, 2nd Edition.
An Alcoholic in the Family by Mary Burton, Faber, 1974.
How to Cope with an Alcoholic Parent by Judith Seixas, Canongate Books, 1980.
How to Control Your Drinking by Dr Miller and Dr Munoz, Sheldon Press, 1983.

Books mentioned in the text:
Peace from Nervous Suffering by Dr Claire Weekes, Angus and Robertson.
Self Help for Your Nerves by Dr Claire Weekes, Angus and Robertson.
How to Stop Worrying and Start Living by Dale Carnegie, Cedar Press.
Making Marriage Work by Dr Paul Hauck, Sheldon Press, 1979.